A Cool Little Book of Meditation

Easy and Unexpected Ways
to Calm and Clear Your Mind and Spirit

By Catherine Kane

A Cool Little Book
Of Meditation

Easy and Unexpected Ways
to Calm and Clear
Your Mind and Spirit

By Catherine Kane

Foresight Publications
Wallingford, Ct.

A Cool Little Book of Meditation- Easy and Unexpected
Ways to Calm and Clear Your Mind and Spirit
© May 2023 by Catherine Kane

I.S.B.N. 979-8-9883057-0-5

Foresight Publications
Wallingford, CT

Table of Contents

Introduction

When I was a child, I had a very active mind.

When I was a teen, my mind became even more active. I often had problems sleeping because my mind was racing. I couldn't get it to slow down enough to drop into slumber.

When I was in college, a hypnosis show came to the campus. I didn't know why, but I felt that it was really important for me to go to it. I begged one of my teachers to be excused from a conflicting class, and he, being a great teacher and seeing that I was serious about this, let me go.

And at the hypnosis show, I had my first experience of what a calm and clear mind felt like. Of altered states.

It was amazing.

And everything changed for me.

That first experience of hypnosis put me on the path which led to a wide variety of meditation and altered states, and what a calm and clear mind could do for me.

It changed my life.

And now I want to put my experience at your service. To show you ways that you can find your own calm and clear mind.

This book is an introduction to meditation and how it works, a collection of different ways to meditate, and instructions on finding the meditation practice that's right for you. It's here to get you started on meditation if you so choose.

Meditation helped make my life better. I hope that it helps make your life better too.

The meditator in me bows to the meditator in you.

Namaste.

Chapter 1
What is Meditation?

So, what is meditation?

The Cambridge Dictionary says that meditation is "the act of giving your attention to only one thing, either as a religious activity or as a way of becoming calm and relaxed." I really like that explanation.

Meditation is found in every culture in every part of the world. Whether it's prayer, or trance dancing, or contemplation, or tai chi, every culture has ways of focusing the mind, finding your center and being present in the moment to get calm, centered and in touch with the Infinite. Your center is that point of experience where your body, emotions and spirit are in balance; and finding and staying in your center supports your health and well-being, feels good, and helps you to have a better life.

Meditation helps us to feel better, get healthier, clear our minds, and get in touch with our spiritual selves. It helps us to make better choices by clearing other thoughts so we can focus on what we need to focus on. It's a little vacation from the rush and multitasking of everyday life. It gets us ready to return to our lives, renewed and refreshed.

And it feels great, too.

The question then isn't whether people should meditate. The question is what kind of meditation works best for each unique person. Since there are lots of ways to meditate, the odds are good that everyone can find their own ways to find their centers.

We've got lots of ways to do that here. You may not like all of them, and that's fine. What's important is seeing if there's one or more that you like that can also fit comfortably into your own life. You need to do you, and this book gives you options for doing that.

Chapter 2
Why Meditate?

Why might you want to meditate?
Studies find that meditation:

- is helpful with emotions such as anxiety, rage, and fear;
- decreases stress, and health conditions associated with stress, such as heart attack and stroke;
- clears the mind;
- decreases high blood pressure;
- bolsters the immune system, supporting more appropriate immune responses.

In short, it does a body good. Better yet, it helps and heals us in body, mind. and spirit.

Besides the mind – body physical benefits, there are other reasons why it's good to meditate.

We live in a world of multitasking. Most of us have multiple things that we're juggling at the same time. Multiple thoughts. Multiple relationships. Multiple projects.

And that's fine, but it comes with a price attached. When we're juggling multiple thoughts and relationships and projects, and always thinking three steps ahead, we can lose track of what's directly in front of us- and that can cause problems. Mistakes. Injuries. Damage to those relationships.

We need the ability to multi task but we also need the ability to focus as well. To be present with what we're doing.

And meditation can help us learn how to focus. To be present in the moment. To put the other things aside for the moment so that we can focus on the task we chose to be present and then to pick up another of those other things and be present for that.

That's a useful skill. Focus is not just useful for

succeeding in the many tasks on our plate. It's also helpful for making well informed, good choices.

When we're in multitasking mode, our minds tend to be crammed full of information and questions:

- What am I going to have for dinner tonight?
- Remember to transfer money and pay this week's bills.
- What do I want to do with my life and how can I do it?

These are all important things, but when you have them and millions of others like them filling up your head and screaming at you, you can easily become distracted and have a hard time being present with the choices that you need to make as well as with making good choices.

Meditation can help. It can teach you how to focus and screen out all of the other things until you've settled this particular one. By doing that, you can access the information that you need and make better choices.

This is also a useful skill.

Finally, the ability to focus is important for energy work.

Some people believe in energy work. Some people do not. Either belief is o.k.- but if you do believe in energy work, then focus is important. Whether you think of it as prayer, magic, manifestation, energetic healing, or just collectively refer to it as energy work, all of it starts with focus and the ability to send your energy in the direction that you want. The better you are at focusing, the better you'll become with your variety of energy work.

Meditation can help you with that.

The ability to calm and clear your mind and spirit will help you put the best effort possible towards working with energy. To focus on your objective and keep your focus there for as long as you need to.

And that's a third reason why you might choose to meditate.

A lot of people don't meditate because they think that it will require too much of them. Several hours a day of meditation. A vegetarian diet. A saintly lifestyle.

Now all of those things are fine, but I'm here to tell you that they're not required. While long periods of meditation are good for you, multiple medical studies have shown that meditation for as short as three to five minutes at a time can have a positive effect on your health in body, mind, and spirit...

You heard me...

Three to five minutes...

And that's not hard to find. That's:

- One commercial;
- One stop light;
- Less time than standing in line at the grocery.

Just about anyone can find 3-5 minutes. I can. You can. So, let's look at meditation and how it can fit into your life.

We're going to look at a lot of different ways to meditate.

First, we'll start by taking a closer look at the basics of meditation and how it works.

That's in the next section. See you there.

Meditation-
the Basics

Chapter 3
Meditation and Your Brain

You can sit in a lotus position. You can chant. You can focus your thoughts and calm the "monkey mind."

But, if we want to understand meditation, we first need to look at our brain waves...

Brain waves are made up of energetic vibrations at different speeds. Let's get to know the different levels.

- At Gamma, you're actively processing information learning, concentrating and solving problems.
- At Beta, you're alert and wide awake but paying attention to everything that's going on around you. A conscious state of multitasking, good for thinking, concentration, and doing things.
- At Alpha, you're more focused and you ignore input that you don't need. Relaxing and pleasant, great for creativity, visualization, and stress reduction.
- At Theta, you're in a "twilight state" between waking and sleeping. Helpful for meditation, intuition, and memory. Good for reprogramming your beliefs, especially unconscious ones.
- And at Delta, you're in deep, restful sleep. Essential for health and healing.

Different activities go better with different waves. Different kinds of meditation use different brain waves, and help us access the brain waves we need for other tasks more easily. Most meditation falls into alpha state, theta state or on the edge between the two.

Meditation can be chanting, or mantras, or the lotus position. It can also be walking, or breathing, or doing the dishes. Anything you do that takes you into that "altered state" can be a meditation, with all the benefits.

What's meditative state feel like? How do you know

when you're in that state? Let's look at that next.

Meditation takes us into an "altered state" – an "asleep but awake" state different from our usual condition. Different altered states are helpful for things like creativity, stress reduction, intuition or healing.

Altered states are also known as "hypnotic states" or "meditative states." That's because the brainwaves active in meditation are also active in hypnosis or self-hypnosis.

How do we know if we're in altered state, anyway? What's it feel like? Surprise. You've probably already experienced it, not once, but many times...

- Ever gotten so into a TV program that you lost track of what's going on in the room around you?
- Ever gotten lost in your thoughts and completely missed what the person talking to you said?
- Ever "jumped" when something happened in the theatre because you were so focused on a movie?
- Ever ridden in a car from one place to another and not remembered the trip in between?

These are all examples of everyday "altered states". Your brain was so focused on one thing that it filtered out all others. Altered states tend to:

- include singleness of thought;
- shut down mental multitasking;
- lead to an experience that's calming, relaxing and feels really good.

The practice of focus can take you into a meditative state. The practice of relaxation can, too.

But before we go there, we need to get to know the "monkey mind".

Chapter 4
The Monkey Mind

In everyday life, our thoughts are racing most of the time. This is especially true if you're multi-tasking. You're always thinking three steps ahead. Your head is full of what you're doing, what you're going to be doing and the two steps in between (and don't get me started on thoughts of the past that come drifting in as well…)

Your mind is always chattering. Some meditation practices even refer to this as "the monkey mind" (with good reason.)

Meditation helps to calm the "monkey mind"- to give us a space when we're not constantly thinking. A rest for the mind. This is one of the reasons that it's so soothing, restful and calming.

That's not always easy. If you're used to your mind chattering all of the time, it won't always just stop because you tell it to.

You're trying to meditate – to soothe your mind and smooth out your chi. And then these darn thoughts keep interrupting, like bratty little children tugging at the skirts of your mind.

- What are you going to have for dinner tonight?
- Is my friend mad at me?
- And my personal favorite-

  - "Gosh, I'm getting good at meditation and focusing on my breath!"
  - "DARN! I just lost my focus congratulating myself! I'm so bad at this!"
  - "DRAT! I'm still distracting myself from my focus!"
  - "RATS! There I go again!"

And so on.

You can distract yourself pretty well by beating yourself up for being distracted.

So, how do we deal with the monkey mind? How do we get back to that calm, cool meditative state, rather than getting absorbed by thoughts of the bills due next week, what's on TV, and the political scandal of the day?

You can't fight those thoughts. If you try and push them away or not think them, you'll trigger resistance, and they'll come back bigger and stronger than before.

- (Don't think about a polar bear!)
- (Did you think about the polar bear?)
- (Well, that's the kind of thing I mean…)

If distracting thoughts intrude, we'd do better to acknowledge them but tell them "not now."

Just stay calm. Don't beat yourself up for being distracted for a moment. It happens to everyone.

Instead think "I see that I'm thinking about Great Aunt Ethel, and I am now returning my thoughts to my breathing."

And go back to your meditation.

There's another way to approach distracting thoughts. You can just let them drift on through.

When a distracting thought comes (and come they will, especially when you're just getting started), acknowledge it. Say "oh, there's a thought…"

Then let it drift on through your mind and out the other side. Pay it no mind. Return your attention to your focus.

I like to think of these thoughts as being like fluffy clouds, drifting across the bright blue sky of my mind.

Sounds silly, but works well. and who could ask for

more than that?

When the monkey mind chatters (and it will), remember, don't fight it. That'll only make it cling on tighter. Just acknowledge those thoughts and put them aside. They'll be there when you finish meditating if you still want them.

Let them go.

And give your mind a break from the chatter.

Next, let's look at visualization and guided meditations.

Chapter 5
Visualizations and Guided Meditations

Visualizations and guided meditations are two different ways to meditate. They use specific methods to get to a meditative state and use that state to accomplish things. Some meditations use some or all of these techniques. Others do not.

Let's take a closer look at how they work.

Visualization is a type of meditation where you create a picture, image or experience in your mind. It's great for skills acquisition and for manifestation work, amongst other things.

Even though it's called visualization, it's about more than sight. You need to include as many senses as you can in a visualization. As an example, in a visualization about riding a horse, you need to include things like:

- What the horse and the area you were riding through looked like;
- The sounds you could hear as you rode;
- What your body felt like as the horse ran;
- The smell of the fresh air;

(I can't think of any decent way to get taste in here, but if you can, include that, too.)

The more senses you include and the more vivid you make them, the stronger the visualization will be and the more it can do for you.

It's also important to put yourself in the visualization, preferably in the middle of what's happening. For example, I heard a story of a man who wanted to manifest a particular kind of sports car, so he did a visualization. Sure enough, one turned up.

His neighbor bought one.

So make sure to put yourself in the visualization.

Visualizations are also used to help people learn or keep skills. Professional athletes visualize themselves running faster and jumping further, or dunking a basketball. Public speakers visualize themselves giving a great speech and answering questions easily. I've even heard stories of prisoners of war visualizing playing golf while captive, to retain their skills.

It works. They've done studies and they find that people who visualize doing things well improve that skill better than by using practice alone.

If you want to learn things or do things well, one way to do that is to visualize it. It's a technique worth trying.

In a guided meditation, you listen to a story which takes you into a meditative state. It may also help you to do things like:

- Relax;
- Heal;
- Get the answer to a question;
- Access your creativity;
- Get in touch with your intuition;
- And other things like that.

The guide is what makes it a guided meditation. That's someone who tells you the story that guides your thoughts.

The guide can be:

- Someone running the meditation live;
- A recorded voice on an audio or video recording.

You can even create your own guided meditations, recording them and listening to them when you want to have that meditation experience.

This book includes scripts for guided visualizations. My permission is granted to the owner of this book to make a recording for personal use while meditating. Recordings may not be made for commercial purposes. No other part of this book may be reproduced or transmitted in any form, or by any means, electronic or mechanical, including photocopying, recording or by any information storage and retrieval system, without written permission from the author, except for brief quotations in a review.

Some guided meditations are completely structured- they walk you through all the steps of a story. Some combine some guidance with choices. You may be told that you see a place that is relaxing to you or that you receive a gift. Your intuition and unconscious mind then fill in the details.

Guided meditations are good for all of the standard meditation goals. They can also be used for specific goals like:

- Easing pain;
- Supporting healing;
- Getting you in touch with your creativity or your psychic senses;
- Answering questions;
- Getting in touch with spirit guides or totems;

And many other specific goals.

There are lots of pre-made guided meditations out there – on tapes, on line, in classes. If you want, you can create your own for your own specific needs.

Just remember:

- Know what your goal is for the meditation.
- Have a story that supports your goals.
- Start with a relaxation to help you get into a state of meditation.
- Leave yourself enough time to meditate. What enough time means is what works for you. Don't rush.
- Finish with a call to come back out of relaxation and to wake up.

…And speaking of goals, if you want to build your own guided meditation or visualization to support your own goals, there's a couple of steps.

- Know what you're trying to do.
- Think of a good symbol for that. (If you want to have more energy, you could have a beam of light that fills you with energy, or a colorful knob which helps you turn your energy up. If you want to concentrate better, maybe a "concentration" button or special glasses that help you focus.)
- Create a story that puts you together with your symbol.
- Start with a relaxation, then go through your story and end with coming back to your body, so that you're awake and aware.
- Don't rush. Give yourself time to meditate.

There are a couple of detailed guided meditations later in this book. (Light in the Forest and The Magic Tablet.) You can use them as visualizations or guided meditations.

If you record them and listen to the recording, you're using them as guided meditations. If you use your imagination without a recording, that's a visualization.

Either way, they can be helpful tools that can help you calm your mind, find your center, and do other useful things.

Visualizations and guided meditations are good for all of the regular meditation goals. They can help to:

- Calm you down;
- Manage stress;
- Help you relax;
- Improve your focus so you can learn and do things better;
- Focus your mind so you can make better decisions;
- Calm down the monkey mind.

They're also good for other things like:

- Learning something;
- Supporting skill improvement;
- Helping you to answer questions;
- Accessing your intuition;
- Manifestation work.

There's a lot of ways that you can improve your life using visualizations and guided meditations. It's worth trying different types to see what works best for you.

Chapter 6
Ready, Set, Meditate

Meditation doesn't have to be done in a zen setting or elaborate eastern temple. Meditation can be done anywhere and at any time- at the kitchen sink, in a grocery store, on your lunch break.

That being said, since you're learning to calm your mind and clear distractions, it'll be easier if you do what you can to cut down on distractions while you're learning. Later on, we'll look at meditation in your daily routine.

Before you start, set things up to minimize distractions. Pick a time when people are less likely to need you. Silence phones. Turn off the TV. Draw the drapes so you're not distracted by things outside. Minimize sounds, with the possible exception of calm new age music or environmental sounds. (The sound of waves or a breeze can be very helpful.)

You don't need to sit in a lotus pose on a pillow on the floor. Sit comfortably. (If a muscle locks up mid-meditation, it'll mess with your serenity. Trust me- I know.) It's often better to keep arms and legs uncrossed, so that they don't go to sleep.

Position is everything.

If your joints are stiff and sitting on the floor is hard, by all means, sit in a chair. You can also lie down if you like. (If lying down with your eyes closed is likely to lead to snoring, better to sit.)

Some people have a tendency to relax so deeply that they go to sleep when they meditate. The term for this is "somnambulism" (which is a term that's also used for sleep walking, but a different use for the word.) Going that deep is not necessarily a bad thing, but it can stop you from getting conscious feedback from meditating when you want it.

Somnambulists often go so deep that they can't remember what they heard or what they experienced when they're in a meditative state. Some folks also call this meditation amnesia.

It's worth noting that, even if you're a somnambulist, you will snap right out of meditative state if a person or a recording tries to program you for something that goes against your beliefs. (I have experienced this personally.)

If you're a somnambulist, you may need slightly different preparation for meditation. You'd probably do better to meditate sitting upright rather than lying down because being laid out flat makes you more likely to fall asleep. Sit supported in a comfortable chair with arms to keep from falling over or out of the chair.

If you want to decrease how deep you go, try holding something slightly heavy in one hand. If you start to go too deep, your hand will relax and the weight will start to drop out of your hand, triggering you to wake up slightly and hold onto the weight again.

You're developing a feel for balance between going out like a light and not getting deep enough to get into a meditative state and stay there for a while. That balance point is what will give you the most benefits from meditation, and the more that you do it, the easier it will be to get there and stay there for the amount of time that you need.

Start with an environment that supports your calm, and now we're ready to meditate…

A
Meditation
Buffet

Chapter 7
Just Breathe

Let's start with one of the most basic but most useful meditation techniques of all. Let's start with breathing.

Find a time where you're unlikely to be interrupted. Position yourself comfortably. If you're concerned about meditating for a certain amount of time, set a timer, but use one that doesn't make noise that will distract you while you meditate.

Then just focus on your breath.

Feel yourself breathe in, and breathe out, and breathe in again. Keep your attention on your breathing. This is harder than it sounds.

At first, you may find thoughts jumping in to interrupt. We're all so used to multi-tasking that many of us have problems with simply focusing on one thing at a time (even if it feels good and will do us good.)

You may find your list of things to do today, and old grudges, and thoughts like "This is foolish.", "Oops, I got distracted from my breath by thinking. I blew it.", and "Drat, there I am, thinking again!" popping up.

That's the monkey mind talking. Don't fight these thoughts. Just return your focus to your breathing without judging yourself.

You'll find this feels really good after a while. Very restful.

Focus on your breathing for whatever time you have. (5 minutes; 10; whatever.)

Then open your eyes, and go forth to face the day.

That's it. Easy peasy- but with practice, this will help you clear your mind with ease.

Chapter 8
Breathe and...

In the last chapter, we did a simple breathing meditation. Let's build on that.

Find your quiet spot and settle yourself comfortably. Close your eyes.

Just breathe. Breathe in. Breathe out. Breathe in. Breathe out.

Focus on your breathing. Once you're keeping your attention on your breathing, let's add something.

As you breathe out, set your intention that you're breathing out stress. As you breathe in, picture breathing in calm energy.

Out, stress. In, calm. Out stress. In, calm.

Feel the stress gradually leaving your body and your body filling up with calm energy. Feel how good that feels.

When you're ready, open your eyes.

You can do this with other things besides stress and calm. You can:

- Breathe out pain and in health.
- Breathe out fear and in strength.
- Breathe out distraction and in calm focus.

What you choose to work with is up to you. This is a great way to let go of things you don't want and bring in things you do.

So take a deep breath- and let's move on to the next meditation.

Chapter 9
A Body Scan

In the last two chapters, we worked with simple breathing meditations. Now we're going to add another step to that- a body scan.

Take a deep breath in. Hold it for a moment, and then breathe out fully, releasing any stress or negativity with the breath. Repeat three times.

Keep breathing. As you breathe, mentally go through each part of your body in turn, looking for parts that are tense or tight, such as neck, jaw or back. Start at your toes, then your feet and move through the parts of your body in order.

When you find a part of your body that's tense, stop and take a deep breath. Relax that part of your body as you breathe out, and then take another deep breath, picturing that part of your body being filled with protective and healing light.

When you've gone through your body and relaxed any tight parts, it can be helpful to move your body or even to wiggle to move muscles out of cramped positions.

Take one more deep breath, and feel yourself calm, centered and at peace.

This is not always as simple as it sounds – but the more you practice, the better you'll get at it.

A breathing meditation or a body scan is a great thing to do when you're waiting- waiting for an appointment, standing in line, waiting for a meeting to get started. Rather than feeling stressed or impatient, you can take that moment to breathe, and relax and meditate your way back to balance. If you feel stressed because you have some place to go, do what you can to relax. Accept that what you're waiting for will happen fast as it can and no faster. Holding onto stress won't change that. It only makes you feel bad. So, take another deep breath and breathe out as much stress as you can let go of.

When you're waiting, you're present. It's much better to be present with peace than with frustration.

Chapter 10
Let Tension Go

Because we live in a busy world, we tend to build up tension. Many times, that tension settles in our muscles and joints.

The shoulders. The jaw. The neck. The back. Any part that's part of you can get tense and tight and painful when you're stressed. Meditation can help with that.

Pick a time when you'll be free from interruptions for a few minutes or more. Put yourself in a comfortable position, sitting or lying, with your arms and legs uncrossed (so that they won't go to sleep.)

Close your eyes.

Start by doing some breathing to relax. As you feel your body start to relax, begin to gently go through the different parts of your body, starting with your toes and working your way upwards.

Where are you holding your tension? Your neck? Your back? Your jaw?

When you find a part of your body that's tense, stop there and breathe. Tense that tight muscle, as tight as you can. Hold it that way for a moment.

Then relax it, breathing deeply. Picture yourself breathing light into that part of the body – light that fills it, heals it and lets it relax.

Be aware of that part of you as it relaxes. See how good it feels? That's how it's supposed to feel. Make a note of this feeling. The next time it starts to get tense, you'll be more aware of it, and know that you need to do some more relaxation.

Once that part of your body relaxes, move on to the next. If a part of your body is holding tension, tense it as much as you can, hold and then relax it.

And, when your time is up and your body is relaxed, open your eyes.

This is a simple but effective technique to decrease stress and relax muscular tension. You can do your whole body, or if you've only got a little time, you can focus on the parts of your body where you tend to carry your tension. By doing this practice, you'll be more aware of the specific places where your stress tends to hang out and you can target them specifically.

Basic body scan or tense and relax- either way, it's good for your head and good for your body as well. (Tense muscles not only hurt but are also more vulnerable to injury.)

So, go ahead. Relax!

Chapter 11
Listen

Meditation is about focusing on one thing and letting everything else go for a while. We do this to:

- take a break from multi-tasking;
- still the "monkey mind's chattering;"
- calm the mind.

Sometimes, meditation is about a specific practice, like breathing meditations. Sometimes it's not. Sometimes, it's about being totally present in what you're currently doing. Not thinking about what's for dinner, or what you want to do on the weekend, but being totally present and focused on what you're doing, whether it's scrubbing a bath tub, doing an exercise, or tickling a child.

It's about being present in the moment.

Settle yourself in a comfortable position, sitting or lying down. (If you think you might fall asleep, sitting is better.)

Close your eyes and take a deep breath. Hold it for a moment, then breathe out, feeling tension and stress leave your body with the breath. Repeat at a leisurely pace until you're feeling calm and centered.

Once you're feeling calm, keep your eyes shut and start to listen to what you hear around you.

What do you hear?

Do you hear:

- the sounds of people around you, or vehicles passing by?
- the sounds of nature?

- the environmental sounds of your surroundings, like the humming of lights, or the gurgle of water in pipes in the wall?
- The sounds of your breathing or your heart beating?

We tend to screen out many of the sounds around us, unless it's a sound that's important. By focusing on them as opposed to screening them out, we can use these sounds as ways to focus and go inwards, and find our center.

Don't make this into a test or a challenge. Just relax, and focus on the sounds around you.

- Can you tell what you're hearing?
- Once you do, can you start to play with this?
- Can you focus on one sound to the exclusion of others?
- Can you shift your focus from one sound to another?
- Can you hear the silence that lies between the sounds and that connects them?

Spend a little time with the sounds and the silence that lies between. And, when you're ready, take a deep breath, return your focus to your body and open your eyes again...

When you've got a moment, spend it with the sound and the silence, and renew your spirit.

Chapter 12
A Meditation Snack

In modern society, we're often on the run. We get a whole lot of stuff done, but we also lose the ability to be present with what we're doing now. If you're always thinking too fast and too far, that can just wear you out.

As we noted in the previous chapter, one kind of meditation is simply being totally present with what you're doing at the moment. Putting multitasking and thinking ahead aside for a while and really being there with what you're doing now in the moment, whether chanting, or exercising, or playing with a bunny.

Being present helps to still the chatter of the monkey mind, and build an inner calm, which is pleasant, relaxing, and healing. One time that you can do this is while eating.

Choose a time and place for your eating meditation where you won't be interrupted. Turn off the phone, and position yourself where folks won't come by every few seconds wanting to chat or for you to find their lost sneaker.

Choose an item of food to focus on. An orange or apple is traditional, but you can do this with any type of food, even a cookie or a veggie burger.

Put aside any worries, planning, or thinking about the next three things on your to-do list. This is just a little meditation, and all of those things will be there when you get back from it.

Start by focusing on the food that you are holding in your hand.

What does it feel like?

- Is it heavy or light? How heavy? ("pretty heavy" or "kinda light" are legitimate responses.)
- What is its texture?
- Is it hard, or soft? If soft, try "squishing" it a bit, to see what that feels like.

28

Look at your food. Turn it over, and look at it from all sides. What does it look like?

- What color is it?
- Is it a solid color or lots of different ones?
- Look closely enough at it so that you would be able to identify it from out of others of its type.

How about sound? Is your food:

- Crispy like a chip?
- Crunchy like good french bread?
- Thumpable, like a melon?

Bring your food up to your nose now, and smell it. Is the smell:

- Sweet?
- Tangy?
- Rich?
- Bland?

And now finally, it's time to taste. Take a small nibble of your food and hold it in your mouth for a moment. Really focus on the flavor and how it feels on your tongue. Start to chew, and notice how the experience changes for you.

The more deeply you focus on your food, the more your mind will calm and your stress will lessen. Meditation is good for your health in general, but a food mindfulness meditation like this can also help develop better eating habits. That can help with indigestion and weight.

Spend as little or as much time being present with your food as you like. If distracting thoughts come up, and the monkey mind begins to chatter, you know how to deal with this.

So, enjoy your mindfulness snack, and have a better day.

Chapter 13
The Art of Meditation

Getting in touch with your creative side is another good way to meditate. As an example, coloring is very popular for adults these days, and we can use that as a meditation too.

Prepare for a coloring meditation as you would for other kinds of meditation.

- Clear your time;
- Minimize distractions;
- Gather what supplies you need to color, so that you're ready to focus.

Start by relaxing. Take deep breaths or tense and relax your muscles.

Give yourself permission to focus on coloring without being distracted by anything else.

Start coloring. Pay attention to this and only this.

- You can focus on the colors and how they look together.
- You can focus on the experience. How does the pencil feel in your hand? How does it feel when you color lightly? How does it feel when you press down harder?
- You can focus on the emotions that the act of coloring make you feel.

The important thing is to color and let focusing on coloring clear your mind and help you find your center.

Any act of creativity can be a meditation. Creating something beautiful is another way to still and focus your mind and find your center. Try finding peace in the act of creating.

Chapter 14
Sound and Meditation

We've talked about how meditation works by focusing on one thing at a time in order to calm your mind for a bit. Sound is one thing that can help you do this in lots of different ways. Not every type of sound works for every person but most people can find one or more types of sound that calm their minds. Let's look at a few types of sound to help you find what works for you.

There are a lot of audio meditations that are available online and off. Online, you can search for:

- Meditation videos,
- Guided meditations,
- Nature meditation videos,
- Or list the specific kind of meditation that you're looking for.

You'll find a lot to choose from.

The least intrusive type of audio meditation is white noise. White noise is a continuous background sound which tends to induce a focused or altered state.

Everyday noise tends to be both intermittent and somewhat random, and an unexpected noise can distract you and break your concentration. An ongoing background of white noise covers those unexpected sounds and helps you to stay focused.

White noise can be sounds or music. It's usually played at a low volume, one where you can hear it if you try to but don't usually focus on it.

I think of it as an auditory cushion for your mind.

Environmental sounds are one variety of white noise. The sounds of a burbling stream, rain on the roof, the surf on a beach or a gentle wind blowing can both cover up intermittent every day sounds and ease you into a meditative state.

There are lots of recordings of different kinds of sounds of nature that can sooth and clear your mind.

There are also tapes of other sounds that support different levels of specific brain waves. These sounds use a process called brainwave or neural entrainment to help lead your brain waves into levels which are good for different tasks, such as learning, focus, meditation, or sleep.

Sound is made up of vibration. So are brainwaves. The theory of entrainment says that when you put two kinds of vibrations together, they will gradually shift to be more like each other. At that point, sounds that are in harmony with a specific brain wave state can make it easier to shift your brain waves to that state.

Like other kinds of white noise, these recordings should be played at a low volume as back ground sound to gradually slide your brain waves into the levels you're looking for.

White noise, environmental sounds and entrainment are three examples of using sound to help you move into altered states. Guided mediations are ways to drop into meditation for more specific purposes.

A guided meditation is a process of audible direction to accomplish a task, such as to support healing, to answer questions or to access your intuition. As opposed to background sound, you actively listen to it, so it's not something that you can have playing while you do something else. (No driving or using heavy machinery while you listen to this.)

It's best to minimize distractions while you listen to a guided meditation. Turn off the phone. Send your roommate to the movies. Some guided meditations will ask you to use head phones.

Put yourself in a comfortable position, sitting or lying down. Legs and arms should be uncrossed. (Otherwise, they'll fall asleep.)

The voice on the meditation will first ease you into relaxation and altered state, then walk you through a story that will help you to accomplish your objective, and then finally bring you back to a normal waking state of awareness. We have examples of guided meditations later in this book.

Some meditations are more structured. They'll tell you things like "You feel more energetic." or "You find it easier to do the things that you need to do." Some leave spaces for you to listen to your own inner wisdom, such as encouraging you to read a magic book or talk to a special guide and then asking what you learn from them. Either approach is valid and can help you to get answers or develop new skills. Which one you choose is totally up to which one you prefer.

It can be helpful to keep a record of what insights or information you get from guided meditations. As you return from altered state, information can get lost, so it's good to write it down right away.

Before we wind up this topic, I want to touch briefly on audio techniques that use meditative techniques and add them to other practices.

Subliminal recordings and hypnosis programs both use different kinds of meditative relaxation to take you into altered states. In these altered states, it's easier for you to make changes that you're ready for in your beliefs, both conscious and unconscious.

This can more directly affect the choices you make, the things you do, and something called the "mind – body connection" which can affect your health and physical well-being.

The mind - body connection works on the premise that what we believe affects our body and our body affects our beliefs. In other words, what you believe shapes what is true for you.

By changing beliefs that limit us to ones that support our health and happiness, we can change our lives for the better.

And subliminal and hypnotic programming can help us do that.

Now we're getting to the level of meditative sounds that give you more specific directions- of subliminal recordings and of hypnosis. At this point, it's time to look at ways of presenting these directions. This is called voice.

Subliminal recordings and hypnotic recordings can be given in either the permissive voice or the authoritative voice.

The permissive voice tends to be more gentle. It says things like "you may find this" or "you can." It gives you options that you can choose to take or choose not to. It gently leads you into a new belief and is less likely to stimulate internal resistance. If you don't like being told what to do, permissive voice may be a better choice for you

The authoritative voice is more forceful. It says things like "you will find this" and "you do this." It's more powerful overall for creating change quickly than the permissive voice but it also is more likely to trigger internal resistance. Overcoming your own internal resistance can take more time and effort than using a gentler permissive approach.

It's up to you to choose the method that works best for you.

If you're comfortable with following directions (particularly directions that you have chosen for yourself in the first place), authoritative voice will be fine for you and will get you faster results. If you tend to resist following directions, you'll do better with permissive voice. (It won't be as fast as authoritative voice but you'll spend less time wrestling with yourself so the results may work to be about the same amount of time or less with less annoyance factor.)

When we want to make a change, sometimes it goes smoothly. Because change can be hard or scary, sometimes we'll develop resistance and cling to our old beliefs though. At that point, choosing the better voice for our unique selves can help to make our change easier.

Subliminal recordings are designed to reprogram your unconscious beliefs to ones that are more beneficial to you and to clear out dysfunctional beliefs in the process.

They usually consist of a series of repeated affirmations with a covering level of sound, nature noise or music. Once again, you play it as background sound.

Many subliminal recordings include a list of the messages that are being shared. If yours does, you can check it to see if you're comfortable with that specific program or whether you need to look for a different one.

It's worth noting that, while most subliminal programs can change your beliefs if you're ready to change, your beliefs can't be changed against your will. If you find yourself feeling uncomfortable when listening to a specific subliminal, that's a pretty good sign that this particular recording is not a good fit for you and you should look for a different subliminal.

And then there's hypnosis.

As opposed to the layer of cover sound in a subliminal recording, hypnosis has its' message right out in the open. A hypnotic program may be accompanied by sound or music, but you can clearly hear the message.

In hypnosis, the hypnotist first uses their voice to ease you into a meditative state, gives you suggestions that can help you change your beliefs or behavior from dysfunctional to something that supports your health and happiness more and concludes by bringing you back to an alert, beta wave state. The voice used can be authoritative or permissive.

And, just as it is with subliminals, hypnosis can help you to make changes that are difficult for you but it cannot be used to control you or to compel you against your will. From personal experience, if you go into an altered state and someone tries to give you a suggestion that you're not comfortable with, you will snap out of altered state and back to an alert state immediately. (This happened to me once in a hypnosis class, and, while it was not a good time, in retrospect it was good because it gave me direct experience that hypnosis was safe and that it couldn't be used to mess with my head.)

Just as authoratative voice subliminals are stronger than permissive voice subliminals, hypnosis is more powerful than subliminals overall. They're all just tools so that you can choose the option that suits your unique needs best.

There are plenty of audio meditations available to sample or buy on the internet. Some groups offer free samples you can try before you buy to see if they suit you. Some offer free meditations in exchange for doing things like signing up for email. Some are only available if you purchase them.

I tend to like the free samples to start out with. No meditation is a perfect fit for everyone, and being able to try them first lets you find the ones that suit you as opposed to rub you the wrong way.

You can also buy copies in new age shops or at alternative health faires. If you take a relaxation or stress management class and they use a recording that you like, it's good to get the name of it so that you can pick it up for your own collection.

These are just a few of the many options available for you online, just to get you started.

Whether you run a recording of nature sounds in the background, take time to listen to a guided meditation, or dive into hypnosis, sound can be a helpful friend when it's time to meditate.

Chapter 15
Meditating in Line

In previous chapters, we've mainly talked about meditations that are done with your mind alone.

Let's look at a different kind of meditation- physical or moving meditation. As one example, let's meditate while standing in line.

Everyone stands in line. At the grocery, at the post office, at a store or restaurant or amusement park. Standing in line is one of the biggest time wasters in every one's life. Unless you meditate while you do it.

While we're standing in line, we're going to do a miniature version of a walking meditation.

Start by moving your feet apart slightly, improving your balance. You can close your eyes if it's safe to do so. You can also do this meditation with your eyes open.

Take a deep breath, breathing out any tension or anxiety as we've done before. (If it's been a tough day, take as many deep breaths as you need.)

Briefly do a quick version of the body relaxation scan. When you find tension in your body, stop and breathe relaxation into it to relax it.

Bring your attention to your feet. Pay close attention to the contact your feet have with the ground – how your body pushes downwards against the earth, and how the earth pushes up against your feet.

Sway gently back and forth. Focus on how the pressure on your body and other sensations shift as different parts of your feet take more or less weight.

When the line permits, take one step forwards. Take the step as s-l-o-w-l-y as you can without the people in line behind you throwing things at you.

Slowly lift one foot and swing it forwards through the air. Place your heel down, paying close attention to how that feels, then s-l-o-w-l-y roll your weight onto your heel, over your arch, and onto the ball of the foot.

Repeat, stepping s-l-o-w-l-y onto the other foot.

As you move onto the other foot, focus on how your first foot pushes off s-l-o-w-l-y with your toes.

Repeat the process with the next step.

Being present in the now – doing a simple action slowly and focusing totally on it can help to still the mind and relax the body.

And you're doing all that while everyone else is wasting their time standing in line.

Clever you...

Chapter 16
Making Life into Meditations

We've been talking about meditation and ways to make little bits of meditation a part of your normal day. We've looked at things like breathing, eating, relaxation, waiting, standing in line, and listening.

Have you thought about making other parts of your day into meditations?

By now, you've probably noticed that one important part of meditation is focusing your attention on a single thought, thing or experience. Focus helps us to relax, calms the monkey mind, and brings us to our centers and the peace that we can find there.

And any activity you can use to create intense focus can be turned into a meditation.

We can certainly find a focus in things we do every day. Whether you're cleaning the bathroom, playing video games, doing dishes, folding laundry, exercising, or doing jigsaw puzzles, almost any basic repetitive activity can also be an exercise in presence, relaxation and meditation.

You do the task that you're doing. You breathe deeply. You relax. You focus totally on what you're doing, on being fully present with it. You pay attention to the sights, the sounds, the sensations of your activity. And you let the acts that fill your day become a meditation.

There are no limits to meditation. The only question is what are you going to bring your peace and presence to today?

Guided
Meditations

Permission to make a recording for personal use

The next two chapters are guided meditations / visualizations.

They are designed to do all of the things that standard meditation does, to support healing in your body, mind and spirit; and to help you to access your inner wisdom and intuition to answer questions that you haven't been able to answer in other ways.

They're different types of guided meditations.

- One of them has all of the meditation spelled out for you and you just follow it.
- The other has spaces that you fill in for yourself with your own intuition.

This gives you two different meditations and also shows you the formats to build your own.

You can:

- review these meditations,
- close your eyes,
- go into altered state and
- go through them;

or you can make a recording of them for your personal use during meditation.

I grant permission to the owner of this book to make a recording for personal use while meditating. (Consider it a gift from me to you.)

Recordings of this book may not be made for commercial purposes. No other part of this book may be reproduced or transmitted in any form, or by any means, electronic or mechanical, including photocopying, recording or by any information storage and retrieval system, without written permission from the author, except for brief quotations in a review.

Chapter 17
Light in the Forest

(This is a guided visualization, where most of the story is set up for you. You can read this and picture it in your head, or you can record it and listen to it while you visualize.)

Close your eyes and relax. Breathe deeply and feel the relaxation sink into every part of you.

Picture yourself in a green, green forest. The trees around you are tall and strong and tower overhead. Here and there, a sunbeam peeks down to the forest floor. The air is crisp and clean and smells wonderful as you breathe in and out, in and out. It's quiet and still except for the little sounds of a living wood, of birds and little animals and green things growing. You feel wonderful and safe in this beautiful place.

You walk along and come to a clearing. You see a woodland pool in the heart of the wood. This pool is full of light, a beautiful fluid light of all the colors that you can imagine.

You dip one finger in and find that it's warm enough to be healing and comforting, and cool enough to refresh you. It feels so good that you decide to go in.

You wade in and as the light covers each part of your body, it feels healthier and more relaxed. Your feet feel great and your legs, your hips, your stomach and your back. Your hands dip into the light and your chest and your shoulders and your neck. Take some time and enjoy this healthy, relaxing, energizing feeling.

At the far end of the pool, you see a waterfall made of light. You decide to wade into the fall and see how that feels. The light falls on all sides of you, on the front and the back and the left and the right. It passes through you, washing away any energy that is negative or unhealthy or that gets in the way of your health and happiness. That unwanted energy is washed away. Your body fills with positive healing light.

When you're ready, you move out from under the falls, feeling healthy and positive and energized. You feel wonderful as you come back out of the pool.

It's time to come back now. At your own speed, become aware of the room, aware of your body, aware of your breathing, and, when you are ready, open your eyes.

And you can carry this feeling of health and positive energy with you into your day.

Chapter 18
The Magic Tablet

(This is a more open visualization. Part of the story is set up for you, and there are spaces left for you to fill in, either in advance or with your unconscious mind as you go along. You can read this and just picture it in your head, or you can record it and listen to it while you visualize.)

This is a visualization for getting answers to questions that you're having problems answering in other ways. Start by deciding on your question.

Close your eyes and relax.

Breathe deeply and feel the relaxation sink into every part of you.

Picture yourself sitting in a comfortable chair in a place that feels comfortable and safe. In your hands is an electronic tablet, one that you've never seen before. It has lots of buttons and controls, but the biggest button is brightly colored and labelled Ask.

Type in your question and press the Ask button. Your answer will appear on the screen in front of you. You may see:

- Words,
- Still pictures,
- Moving pictures,
- More than one piece of information,
- Or any other combination that will give you useful information.

So, what answer did you see?

If you want, you can rewind the answer and view it more than once, to get all the details.

If the answer isn't clear, there's a smaller "Clarify" button that will give you more information. Add any other buttons that you need to make this tablet helpful.

Take all the time you need to absorb the information you receive and figure out what it means to you.

And then, when you're ready, slowly open your eyes and come back to the physical world.

This is an open visualization, where we set up a story that will help you to get in touch with your unconscious mind or your intuition and let them fill in the answers. Your unconscious mind knows more things than your conscious mind does. Your intuition has access to more information than your non-psychic senses. A story like this gives you a way to get in touch with your unconscious mind, with your psychic senses, or with both, so that you can make more informed choices.

Feel free to adapt this meditation into something that works best for you. I chose an electronic tablet, but you could also look into a magical book, an enchanted mirror, a big screen tv or a mystical smart-phone and get the same effect, depending on which is better for you. Choose the image that suits you best and use it to help you get messages from your intuition.

Make this into what works best for you or create other stories that help you to know and do things. The point is to tell a story that supports you and use it to become better informed.

Pulling It
All Together

Chapter 19
A Meditation Plan

We've talked about meditation and about different kinds that may work for you. Your first step is to try different kinds to find the ones you like (and it's worth trying a bunch of them more than once. It sometimes takes multiple times to see what's a good fit for you)

And the next step is to actually do the meditations. They won't give you benefits if you don't get around to doing them. It's easy to mean well but somehow let other things get in the way of meditating.

If you want meditation to make your life better, you have to actually make it happen. For that, it helps to have a plan of ways to make meditation a simple part of your life. If it's easy and natural, it's more likely to get done.

Take a moment or two and think about what your day is like. Where could you fit in a quick meditation or two?

If you're waiting for your computer to boot up, you could do a breathing meditation.

If you're waiting for a ride, you could listen to the world around you.

If you're standing in line at the grocery store, you could do a walking meditation.

If you're having lunch, you could do a meditation snack.

If you're sitting in front of the computer, you could put on some headphones and listen to a guided meditation.

If you're waiting for an appointment or a meeting, you could do a body scan.

Almost any daily repetitive routine can be transformed into a meditation. All you need are relaxation, focus, and a willingness to come to that calm, still center within you, and meditation is there.

Sit back, and give some thought to where meditation might find a place in your life. Have a plan. Build a routine.

It can help to tie meditation to activities that you are already doing regularly. Do a quick breathing practice after you brush your teeth. Do a body scan in the shower.

Give yourself reminders if you need to, to take a little meditation break. I find notes saying "Breathe" in my Dayrunner and taped to my bathroom mirror and on the surround of my computer monitor are very helpful to keep the rest of my life from distracting me.

And think about making the meditation that's right for you a part of your everyday life.

Meditation does a body good. Having a meditation plan can make that happen.

Chapter 20
Looking For More

The journey of a million miles begins with a single step. This book is only a starting point. It's here to let you dip your toes into the river of meditation and get comfy with it.

But there's more out there. Lots more…

The meditations in this book were chosen because:

- They're quick and easy to learn.
- They're quick and easy to do.
- They're time flexible. You can do them for a short time or a long one.
- You can do them almost anywhere.
- Most of them don't need special equipment.
- They're great examples for learning the basics of meditation.
- A lot of them are simple enough that children can do them as well as adults can.

Once you've tried different types of meditation and found out what you like, you may want to check out some more advanced varieties. Here's some ideas on how to do that.

We've looked at the basics of meditation in this book, including some simple meditations. There are many more practices out there, everything from mindfulness to transcendental meditation. More complex meditation can include chanting, mantras, or other types of meditation practices.

If you want to explore the world of more complex

meditations, there are lots of resources online. There are intro classes at health food stores, ashrams or adult education, where you can try something different to see if you like it. You can use basic classes as a way to sample different practices with an informed teacher to answer any questions you may have. This is a great way to see if a specific practice is a good fit for you either now or in the future.

...Or in the future. That's an important thing to think about.

You sample now. You find the practices that work for you. You build a routine that helps you to meditate on a regular basis- and that's great.

But some of those practices will be with you for the rest of your life; and some of them will never be your thing. And some of them are not for you now- but that doesn't mean that they never will be.

It's good to keep that in mind. Use the ones you like, discard the ones you dislike, but keep the ones that aren't your thing in the back of your mind and put away safely for your future needs. It's not unlikely that your needs may change and you will want different types of meditation. It's not unlikely that you may get tired of one kind of meditation and need a break from it. It's not unlikely that, after a while, you may need to grow in a new and different direction.

So be aware that a meditation practice may be predictable but that it can also grow and change just like you can grow and change. When you're finding meditation practices that suit you, don't just sort them into "No" and "Yes". Instead sort them into "No", "Yes" and "Not Yet".

Other varieties of meditation to explore are:

Recorded meditations. As we discussed back in the "sound and meditation" chapter, there are lots of meditative sounds and guided meditations available on the internet. A quick search can help you find more advanced meditations.

Or you can study other types of meditation to learn how to build your own.

Other people's meditations can do a good job of helping you to relax, but a custom built meditation where you incorporate elements that speak to you can be very effective, especially if you record it with your own voice.

Another option is yoga, which combines stretching, breathing and meditation. It's a combination of moving and mental meditation. It's usually calm and gentle stretching, but there are varieties of yoga that are more active too.

Tai Chi, and its little sister, Chi Gung (Qi Gong) are moving meditations that combine slow flowing movements, deep rhythmic breathing, and a calm meditative state of mind. They come originally from China, and are practiced all over the world to help people be strong and healthy in body, mind and spirit.

There are lots of different types of Tai Chi and Chi Gung. If you like physical types of meditation, these might be something that you'd like.

You can learn them from a video or might want to find a teacher.

Finding advanced meditations may mean:

- doing research,
- finding a class, teacher or video,
- spending time practicing so it becomes easy for you.

If you find an advanced option that really suits you, it's worth putting in the time and effort to develop a skill that can help you to be healthier and happier.

Whether you like auditory meditation, visualization, guided meditation or any other variety of meditation, the important part is finding what suits you- what works for your preferences and your life style, and is workable to practice on a regular basis.

A calm and clear mind and spirit decreases stress and supports a healthy body, mind and spirit; quiets the monkey mind so you can focus and make good choices; and feels really good. You deserve the gifts that meditation can bring you.

And now we reach the end of this book and the beginning of your adventure. I wish you well on your journey to a calm and clear mind and spirit, and to healing in body, mind and spirit. I hope you find the meditation that is a perfect match for your own unique self.

Namaste.

Glossary

Alpha waves- (8-12 Hz) quietly flowing thoughts and meditative states. The "power of Now." Being here in the present. The resting state for the brain. Good for overall mental condition, calmness, alertness, mind/ body integration and learning.

Altered state- being in a state of meditation or focus.

Auditory meditation – meditation using sound as a focus.

Being present in the moment – tuning out past and future and focusing exclusively on what is happening now.

Beta waves- (12- 35 Hz) good for being wide awake, alert and focused, multitasking and making decisions.

Brainwaves - communication between neurons within our brains. When slower brainwaves are dominant, we can feel tired, slow, sluggish, or dreamy. When higher frequencies are dominant, we can feel wired, or hyper-alert.

Breath work -meditation involving focusing on your breath.

Body scan - moving your attention through the parts of your body to locate tension or dysfunction.

Delta waves- (0.5 - 4 Hz) deep in dreamless sleep.

Entrainment- using sound to ease your brain waves into levels that support the tasks you want to do.

Gamma Waves (upwards of 35 Hz)- good for actively processing information and learning, concentrating and solving problems.

Guided meditation – a process of using an external source and a story to take you through a meditation process; usually to get information or accomplish a task.

Manifestation work – using visualization or focus to change the nature of reality.

Meditation- giving your attention to only one thing, either as a religious activity or as a way of becoming calm and relaxed.

Meditation snack – meditation by focusing on eating.

Mind - body connection – our beliefs affect our body and our body affects our beliefs.

Monkey mind- a hyper-busy mind which is unable to focus.

Moving meditation – meditation that focuses through physical movement, such as Tai Chi.

Namaste- "I bow to you."

Presence - a focus on what you're currently doing.

Practice – 1) a routine of performing an activity in order to benefit from it or get better at it. 2) to actually do that practice on a regular basis.

Resistance- consciously or unconsciously fighting change in your beliefs.

Setting an intention- determining a goal for what your meditation will accomplish.

Somnambulism – meditating so deeply that you lose awareness of your surroundings.

Somnambulist – someone who goes very deeply into meditation.

Tense and relax – relaxation practice involving tensing tight muscles in order to relax them.

Theta waves- (4 - 8 Hz.) experienced when sleeping more lightly or being extremely relaxed.

Visualization – meditation through picturing yourself having an experience and incorporating as many of the five senses as possible.

White noise - a constant background noise, good for supporting focus and a calm and clear mind.

Zen - a Japanese sect of Mahayana Buddhism that aims at enlightenment by direct intuition through meditation.

Index

This book is dedicated to all of the people that I've met who thought that they couldn't meditate:

- because they thought that it was too hard;
- because their minds wouldn't slow down;
- because they thought that they couldn't focus;
- because they didn't have time to meditate;
- because it took too long;
- because they'd never had any success at it before.

I love you all but you've been misled. You can meditate. You just haven't found the way to meditate that's right for you, yet. You just haven't had the tools that you needed to do that in a way that works for you before this.

And the meditation that suits you best is one of the best ways to resolve all of those reasons that you thought that you couldn't meditate in the first place.

There are lots of different roads to enlightenment. There are lots of different ways to reach altered states. The trick is just to find the one or more that works best for your unique mind and spirit.

And this book is here to help you find your jam.

The meditator in me bows to the meditator in you.

Namaste.

Acknowledgements

Welcome to my thirteenth book, the eleventh book in general circulation. Wow! My itty-bitty publishing empire is growing.

My thanks to my beta readers; Tchipakkan, Carol, Jane, Morgan and Cheryl. Your eagle eyes and your kindness help to make this the best book it can be.

My continuing gratitude to my readers and fellow writers who were kind and patient with me, encouraged me, gently nagged me, and kept me writing. What would I do without you?

If you're new to my books, welcome to my world. Pull up a chair and stay awhile. If you're an old friend, welcome back. I saved a chair for you.

All of my love and gratitude to the people and situations that made me the writer that I am now. I continue to hope that you're not sorry about that.

And, with all of my love, to my husband Starwolf, healer, wise and knowledgeable shaman, professional psychic, multi-talented man of all works and general all round good guy. I write, but I couldn't do it without you, dear.

Catherine Kane was raised by feral storytellers.

She's a teller of tales, a teacher, a poet, a wordsmith and a song wright, a professional psychic, an artist, an enthusiastic student of the Universe, a maker of very bad puns and a medieval re-enactor who spends a fair amount of time at renaissance faires when she isn't hunched over her computer, writing.

She's also a bit of an over-achiever.

Want to know more about her?

Find her on Facebook at
https: / / www.facebook.com / Catherine-Kane-Writes / 134304556668759

Your Notes

www.ingramcontent.com/pod-product-compliance
Lightning Source LLC
Chambersburg PA
CBHW070931280326
41934CB00009B/1835